To the Ec

Hand of the Wind Taijiquan:
Book One.

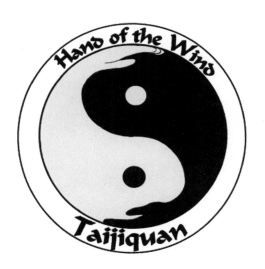

Conrad Robinson

To the Edge of the Cyclone

Hand of the Wind Taijiquan:

Book One.

Basic Principles,
Stances,
Taiji Short Form,
Taiji Feishou Form.

Introduction.

This book is intended to provide an aide-memoire for students attending Hand of the Wind Taijiquan classes. It is not intended to replace competent instruction. The author strongly believes that it is not possible to learn Taijiquan from a book. The intention is that students will be able to use this book to help them remember what they have learnt in class, it is not recommended for students to try to learn new movements from the book.

The book is divided into four sections. Section One provides information on basic principles that we adhere to when training in Hand of the Wind Taijiquan. Section Two provides details of some of the most common stances used within the style. Section Three covers the Taiji Short Form, with photographs and descriptions of the movements of the Form up to number fifty (the end of the sequence: The Edge of the Cyclone). Section four introduces the Taiji Feishou ('Flying Hand') Form.

There is no attempt within this book to explain the theories behind the training. Whilst the author believes that study of Qi theory, Yin and Yang and some understanding of Chinese Medical principles are essential in order to gain a full understanding of the Arts, this book is not intended to be a book of theory. This is intended to be a practical training manual for students attending Hand of the Wind classes where the theory is taught as part of the curriculum.

Contents:

Section One.

Basic Principles.

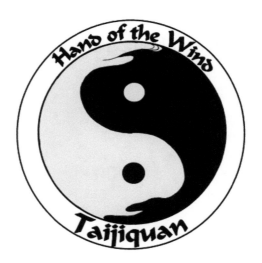

Basic Principles.

Within Hand of the Wind Taijiquan there are certain basic principles which we adhere to throughout our training. These can be broken down into four general aspects – Relaxation, Breathing, Stance and Posture.

This chapter introduces the basic principles within each of these aspects in turn.

Simply adhering to these basic principles of the Art is likely to yield significant benefits to health and well-being. Combining these principles with the exercises and movements of the form, which are designed to encourage the flow of Qi through the body in specific ways, is the way in which the full benefits of the Art can be experienced.

Relaxation.

The most important principle for the art of taijiquan is that of relaxation. We are always aiming to stay as relaxed as possible within everything we do. The concept of 'dynamic tension' is key to this principle of the art.

Dynamic tension means to use the absolute minimum of muscular tension in order to achieve our aim. Therefore, if I were to hold my arm out in front of me I should only be using my muscles to support the weight of the arm – if a snowflake were to land on the arm the extra weight should be sufficient to cause the arm to drop. We can use visualizations to aid us in maintaining this level of relaxation throughout our practice and therefore in life generally.

Breathing.

Within our training there are several exercises we use which can improve the way in which we breathe. There are also aspects of breathing which we should aim to adhere to at all times. Firstly, it is important that we breathe in a relaxed manner, not forcing the breath. Breathing exercises will improve our ability to use more of our lung capacity so that we do not build tension into our bodies through trying to force the breath.

During Qigong breathing exercises, the movement is tied to the breath and therefore it is important to time the movement to the breath. Within Taiji Form training it is better to allow yourself to breathe naturally as you perform the movements and the breath will naturally start to coincide correctly with the movement as your body learns to relax into the moves.

Normally we breathe in and out through the nose, although some breathing exercises will specify breathing in or out through the mouth. At all times it is important to maintain the contact between the tip of the tongue and the roof of the mouth (as if about to make the sound of the letter 'L').

Stance.

The term 'stance' is used to refer to the alignment of the lower body – from the waist down. There are a number of stances we use within Hand of the Wind and they each have names (usually animal names); using the names of the stances allows us to know where our feet and weight should be for each movement.

General principles for stance work involve how we move our feet, where our weight is focused and alignment of the joints of the lower body.

When we move our feet into a new position we place the heel down first and then the ball of the foot before allowing the toes to relax down onto the floor. This ensures a good, relaxed contact between the 'Bubbling Spring' point in the centre of the ball of the foot and the floor.

The weight of the body should be aligned to press down through the 'Bubbling Spring' point in the ball of the foot and not down through the heel.

The pelvis should be aligned so that the tailbone (coccyx) is slightly tucked under the body. This takes pressure off the base of the spine and allows the 'Ming Men' point in the lower back to relax.

The knees should never be locked fully straight so when we refer to a 'straight' leg there is always a slight bend at the knee.

Posture.

Posture is the term we use to refer to the alignment of the upper body – from the waist up. This includes the alignment of the hands and head and so the position of the body within each movement of the Taiji Form is a combination of stance and posture.

As with the legs, the arms should never be locked straight so that even when we refer to a 'straight' arm there is always a slight amount of bend at the elbow. The wrists should not 'lock out' by being bent too far in either direction. Normally the elbows stay below shoulder height except where a specific movement's posture explicitly dictates otherwise. The hands should stay relaxed with the palm slightly 'cupped' to maintain relaxation around the 'Lao Gong' point in the centre of the palm and 'Hegu' on the muscle between thumb and forefinger.

The head should feel as though it were suspended from a point just behind the highest point of the head. This extends the neck and allows the chin to drop slightly.

During most movements the hands stay on their own side of the body and do not cross the centre line. Often when it appears that the hands do pass the centre line it is a turn of the waist rather than movement of the arm that positions the hands.

The elbows and hands rarely come very close in to the body, except where specified by a particular movement. Normally the elbows stay at least a fist width from the body and the hands a full hand span from the body – we often refer to this as the 'critical distance'.

Section Two.

Stances.

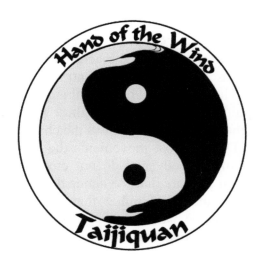

Stances.

General notes for all stances.

In Hand of the Wind Taijiquan we use the term 'stance' to refer to the alignment of the lower body. Stance refers to alignment of the body from the waist down and we use 'posture' to refer to the alignment of the upper body, from the waist up (including arms, hands and head).

In all stances the basic principles must be adhered to, as outlined in the previous chapter.

Key points to remember are:

- Never lock a limb.
- Pelvis should be aligned so that the tailbone is tucked underneath the body.
- Weight is supported by the ball of the foot.
- Toes relax onto the floor.
- Stepping into a stance should be heel-toe.

Within this section photographs are presented showing stances used within the Form. For most of the stances there are also 'footprints' showing the correct foot placement and weight distribution – a black footprint shows a 'weighted' foot, a white footprint shows a foot with little or no weight in it and a grey footprint shows a foot supporting 50% of the body weight.

Eagle Stance.

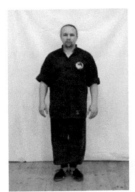 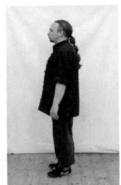

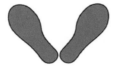

In Eagle stance the heels are together, the legs are straight (but not locked at the knees). The feet angle outwards from the centre line so that there is a maximum angle between the feet of 90° (although less than 90° is more relaxed for most people). The posture is maintained according to the basic principles and the weight is equally distributed between the feet.

Bear Stance.

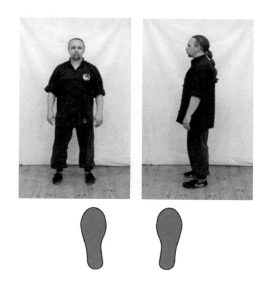

In Bear stance the feet are shoulder-width apart with the feet parallel, both pointing forwards. The knees are 'off-lock' so the legs are a little more bent than in Eagle stance but still with only a minimum amount of bend at the knees. Weight is evenly balanced on both feet.

Riding Horse Stance.

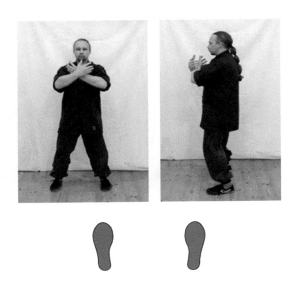

In Riding Horse the feet are wider than shoulder width, with the feet parallel so that the toes are pointing towards the front. The knees are more bent than in Bear stance so the feeling is that you are 'sitting' into the stance. The weight is equally distributed between both feet.

Leopard Stance.

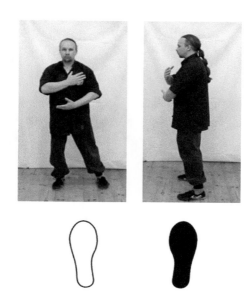

In Leopard the feet are at least shoulder width apart and parallel so the toes are pointing forwards. The weight is directed down into one foot with the knee of the weighted foot bent. The 'light' leg is straight (but not locked) with only the weight of the leg supported by that foot – the majority of the body-weight is supported by the bent leg.

Dragon Stance.

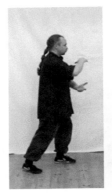 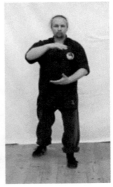

In Dragon the feet are shoulder width apart with one foot advanced to the front. Around 80% of the weight is supported on the front foot which is pointing forwards. The back foot is directed outwards on an angle similar to that in Eagle stance with little more than the weight of the back leg supported by that foot. The front leg is bent and the back leg is straight (but not locked and maintaining the pelvis alignment according to the basic principles). The weight is forward to almost the point where the back heel starts to lift, but not quite, so that the back foot remains flat on the ground. The hips are 'square' facing to the front and the front knee is not extended beyond the toes of the front foot.

Snake Stance.

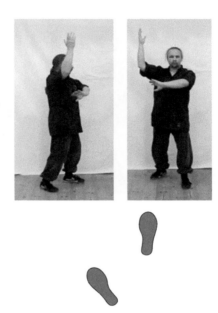

In Snake the feet are shoulder width apart with the hips 'square' facing to the front. The front foot is pointing forwards and the back foot is at an angle similar to Eagle stance. The weight is equally distributed between both feet with both knees bent.

Duck Stance.

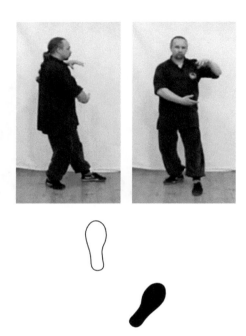

For Duck stance, the feet are shoulder width apart with the front foot pointing forwards and the back foot at an angle. The weight is in the back foot with only the weight of the front leg supported by the front foot. The rear knee is bent with the front leg straight, but not locked. Both feet are flat on the ground. The hips are 'square' facing to the front.

Monkey Stance.

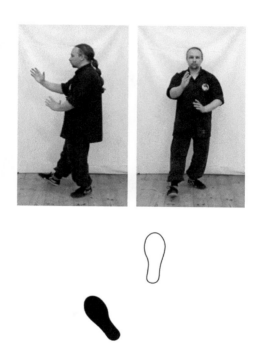

Monkey stance shares many of the characteristics of Duck stance; foot and hip alignment are the same, the back (weight bearing) leg is bent with the front leg straight. In Monkey however, the toes of the front foot are lifted so that only the heel remains on the floor.

Cat Stance.

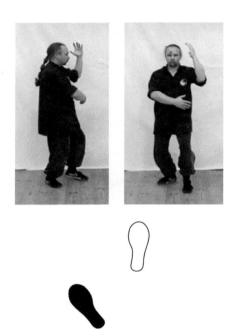

Cat is another stance that shares many characteristics with Duck stance. In Cat stance the front heel is lifted (unlike Monkey where it is the toes that lift). It is important to be aware that the 'Bubbling Spring' point in the centre of the ball of the foot remains in contact with the ground.

Crane Stance.

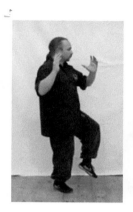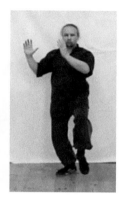

In Crane stance the front foot is lifted off the floor so that all the weight is supported by one foot which is aligned at an angle as in Eagle stance. The front knee is lifted to no higher than would bring the thigh parallel to the floor and the lower leg 'hangs' relaxed from the knee. The front foot relaxes down from the ankle maintaining the feeling of heel-toe as you 'step' into the stance. The standing (weighted) leg is bent at the knee.

Dog Stance.

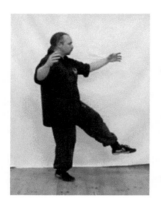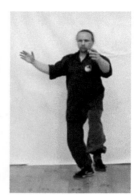

Dog stance is similar to Crane in that it is another stance where the front foot is lifted off the floor. In Dog stance the front foot is extended further forwards than the knee and again relaxes down from the ankle to 'step' heel-toe into the stance. The standing leg is bent and the front leg should be 'off-lock' and at a maximum height of thigh parallel to the floor.

Section Three.

Taiji Short Form.

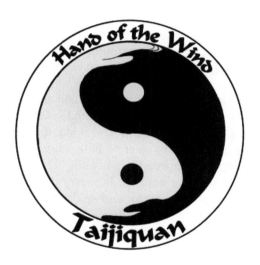

Taiji Short Form.

The full Hand of the Wind Taiji Form contains 42 sequences of movements, for a total of 140 moves. The Short Form comprises the first 15 sequences and the final sequence of the form. For ease of learning we break the form up into numbered 'moves' and the first 15 sequences consist of the moves up to number 50.

It is important to remember that the Form is a means to an end and not the objective of Taiji training. It is a tool which enables us to improve the way in which we use our bodies. The real objective of Taiji training is to take the lessons we learn from our training and apply them to everything we do within our lives.

Taijiquan is a martial art and the health benefits are a side effect of correct martial training. Most people coming to Taiji classes, however, are not seeking martial skill. The beauty of Taiji is that it can cater to both students of the martial and those seeking to improve their health. This book is not intended as a martial training manual, however during classes instructors may use martial imagery to help students to remember and refine their Taiji Forms. Some martial imagery may also be found in descriptions of movements in this book.

For quick reference a table is presented on the following pages showing the stance and direction for each movement. The table assumes an initial position of standing facing South so that when we turn to our right in move 6 we will be facing West. The compass directions are presented for reference only – it does not matter which compass direction you initially face when practicing the form!

Sequence	Move	Stance	Facing
Preparation	Start	Eagle	South
	Prepare	Bear	ˮ
Gather Celestial Energy	1	Eagle	ˮ
	2	Eagle	ˮ
	3	Eagle	ˮ
Play the Guitar	4	Right Dragon	ˮ
	5	Right Monkey	ˮ
	6	Right Dragon	West
Fair Lady Weaving	7	Right Monkey	ˮ
	8	Right Dragon	ˮ
	9	Right Monkey	ˮ
	10	Right Dragon	ˮ
	11	Right Monkey	ˮ
The Crane Exercises its Wings	12	Riding Horse	South
	13	Right Leopard	ˮ
	14	Eagle	ˮ
	15	Eagle	ˮ
	16	Eagle	ˮ
	17	Riding Horse	ˮ
Drive the Tiger Away	18	Left Dragon	ˮ
	19	Right Monkey	ˮ
	20	Right Dragon	South-West
Grasp the Bird's Tail	21	Right Cat	South
	22	Right Dragon	West
Brush Knee and Side Step	23	Right Monkey	ˮ
	24	Right Leopard	South
Repulse the Monkey	25	Left Cat	East
	26	Left Dragon	ˮ

Sequence	Move	Stance	Facing
The Stork is Aroused	27	Left Crane	East
	28	Left Dog	"
	29	Left Monkey	"
	30	Left Dragon	"
The Double Whip	31	Left Snake	"
	32	Left Leopard	South
The Cobra Unwinds	33	Right Leopard	"
	34	Left Dragon	"
	35	Left Cat	"
	36	Right Dragon	West
The Wild Dog Retaliates	37	Right Monkey	"
	38	Left Dog	"
	39	Left Leopard	South-West
	40	Right Dragon	West
The Tail of the Peacock	41	Left Cat	East
	42	Left Dragon	"
	43	Left Monkey	"
	44	Left Dragon	"
Brush Knee and Side Step	45	Left Monkey	"
	46	Left Leopard	South
The Edge of the Cyclone	47	Left Monkey	"
	48	Right Dragon	"
	49	Right Cat	"
	50	Right Dragon	"
Gather Earth's Energy	(1)	Eagle	"
	(2)	Eagle	"
	(3)	Eagle	"

Within this section each movement of the Form is presented with photographs of the end position. Photographs are provided from the 'front' and from one side for each position – the larger photo is from the perspective of a viewer standing to the front at the start of the form; and the smaller image shows the view from the side on which that picture is presented. There is also a description of the movement required to reach that position: this is broken down into stance movement, posture movement and sometimes notes on timing.

Although the movements are separated into stance and posture for convenience within this book, remember that the stance and posture work together and the movements of both the lower and upper bodies must be coordinated correctly. This is another reason why it is not possible to learn these movements from a book and why it is important to learn the moves from a qualified instructor.

Prepare.

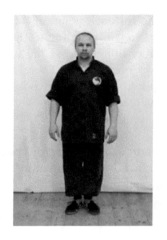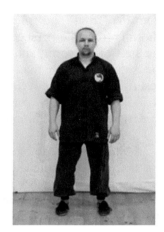

Stance: Bear
Facing: South

Stance movement:

Before starting the movements of the Form, we prepare by stepping from an Eagle stance into Bear stance. This is done by stepping the left foot to the left, placing the heel down and then the toes making sure that the foot is aligned to point forwards. The right foot is then corrected heel-toe to bring the feet into the correct parallel orientation for the Bear stance.

Posture movement:

Arms stay, hanging relaxed, by your sides.

Timing:

Once into Bear stance take a few breaths to allow your body and Qi to settle. When you feel completely still you are ready to start the Form.

Gather Celestial Energy.
Move #1.

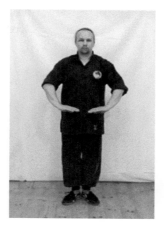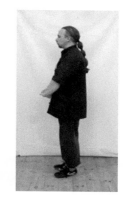

Stance: Eagle
Facing: South

Stance movement:

From the Bear stance correct your right foot (heel-toe) into the correct orientation for Eagle stance. The left foot then draws back in and is placed down heel-toe into the Eagle stance.

Posture movement:

As the feet move into position the hands are brought up and in front of the body with the palms down to finish with the fingertips pointing at fingertips at Tantien level.

Timing:

At the point when both heels touch the hands should be both pointing forwards with the palms down. Then as the weight settles onto both feet the hands turn to fingers pointing at fingers.

Gather Celestial Energy.
Move #2.

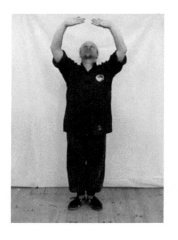 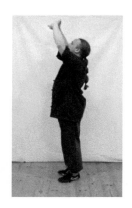

Stance: Eagle
Facing: South

Stance movement:

Stay in Eagle stance.

Posture movement:

Maintaining the Eagle stance, the hands come up in front of the body with the palms facing away, still with fingertips pointing at fingertips. From eye level allow the eyes to follow the hands until looking upwards.

Gather Celestial Energy.
Move #3.

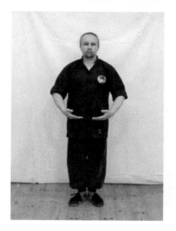 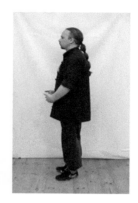

Stance: Eagle
Facing: South

<u>Stance movement:</u>

Still, remaining in Eagle stance.

<u>Posture movement:</u>

The hands return down in front of the body to Tantien height, palms still facing away from the body as they come down, so that the hands are palms down when they reach Tantien height. The eyes follow the hands down until they reach natural eye level. Once the hands reach Tantien height the hands drop from the wrist before turning palms up, fingertips pointing to fingertips.

Play the Guitar.
Move #4.

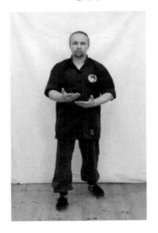 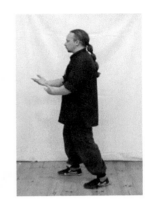

Stance: Right Dragon
Facing: South

Stance movement:

From Eagle stance the weight moves onto the left foot and the right foot steps forwards into position for Dragon stance before bringing the weight forwards onto the right foot.

Posture movement:

The right hand moves across the top of the left hand, still with both palms facing upwards. The hands then move forwards (often described 'as if casting rice from a bowl') with the left hand following the right to finish with the fingertips of the left hand pointing towards the right wrist. Each hand should be just on its own side of the centre-line of the body – a common mistake is to take the right hand too far to the right side of the body.

Play the Guitar.
Move #5.

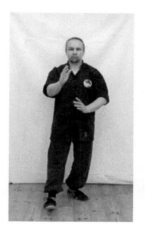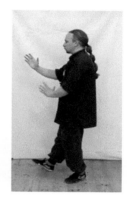

Stance: Right Monkey
Facing: South

Stance movement:

The weight rocks back from the Dragon stance onto the left foot (drawing the foot in a little if necessary) before the toes of the front foot lift to come into Monkey stance.

Posture movement:

The hands open and lift to chest height and roll back into an 'en-garde' position. This movement is often described as coming around a 'ball' – think a rugby ball with the axis angled up and away from you. The palms stay down as the hands move back in towards the body and then at the end of the move they turn thumb edges upwards, with the fingers pointing roughly 45° upwards.

Play the Guitar.
Move #6.

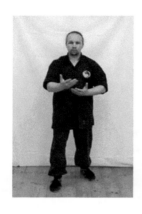 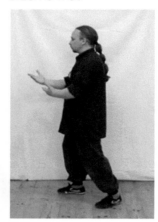

Stance: Right Dragon
Facing: West

Stance movement:

The right foot swings around to the right and is placed down heel-toe. The weight then transfers onto the right foot and as the hips come into alignment for the Dragon stance correct the left foot heel-toe. Consider where you place the right foot to ensure you end in a good Dragon stance and not 'on line'.

Posture movement:

The right hand presses palm down towards the left knee and is followed by the left hand. As the hands come up (palms up) in front of the left hip (right hand over left) the right foot steps. Again, the hand movement can be described as 'casting rice' as in move #4. Hands end with palms up and left hand pointing at the right wrist as in move #4.

Fair Lady Weaving.
Move #7.

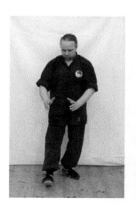 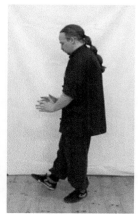

Stance: Right Monkey
Facing: West

Stance movement:

The weight rocks back from the Dragon stance, drawing the foot in a little if necessary and then lifting the toes to come into Monkey stance.

Posture movement:

As in move #5 the hands come up and 'around the ball' before coming back in towards the body. Passing the 'en-garde' position of move #5, the right hand continues down to 'catch up' with the left hand so the hands are palm facing palm in front of the right hip. Towards the end of the move look down to view the foot between the two hands. This position is often referred to as 'holding the rice bowl'.

Fair Lady Weaving.
Move #8.

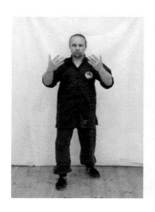 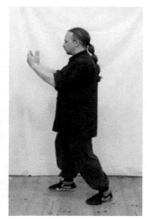

Stance: Right Dragon
Facing: West

<u>Stance movement:</u>

The front foot moves into position for the Dragon stance, stepping forwards heel-toe slightly if required. The weight shifts onto the front foot to come into the Dragon – make sure there is no 'up and down' movement of the body as the weight transfers.

<u>Posture movement:</u>

The hands come up in front of the body with the palms facing in towards the body, describing an arc until they are fingers up in front of the shoulders. The hands move forwards 'pushing with the back of the hands' as the weight shifts into Dragon. The hand movement is often described as being 'over the ball' in this movement.

Fair Lady Weaving.
Move #9.

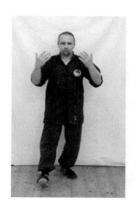 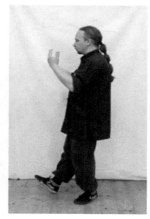

Stance: Right Monkey
Facing: West

Stance movement:

Again, the weight rocks back into Monkey stance, drawing the foot back before lifting the toes if required.

Posture movement:

As the weight shifts back into the Monkey stance the hands return 'under the ball' back to palms facing inwards towards the shoulders.

Fair Lady Weaving.
Move #10.

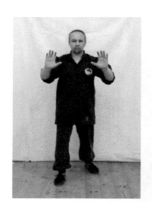 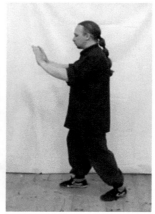

Stance: Right Dragon
Facing: West

Stance movement:

Stance movement is essentially a repeat of move #8, coming forward into Dragon stance again.

Posture movement:

As you settle into the Monkey stance at the end of move #9 the hands start to turn to face palms forwards in front of the shoulders. The movement of each hand is as if they are rolling around two 'balls' held in front of the shoulders. This changes the direction of the circle so that, as you come forward into Dragon 'pushing' with the palms, the hands come 'under the ball'.

Fair Lady Weaving.
Move #11.

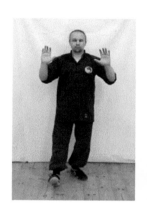 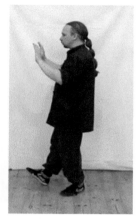

Stance: Right Monkey
Facing: West

Stance movement:

Again, stance movement is essentially the same as move #9 with the weight shifting back into Monkey stance.

Posture movement:

As the weight shifts back into Monkey the hands return 'over the ball' to finish with the palms facing outwards in front of the shoulders.

The Crane Exercises its Wings.
Move #12.

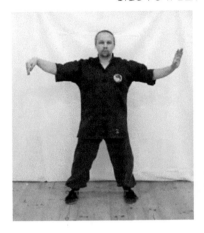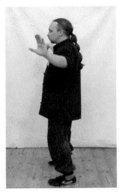

Stance: Riding Horse
Facing: South

Stance movement:
The right foot turns, pivoting on the heel 90° to the right, to finish pointing south. The weight shifts across to enable the correction of the left foot into a parallel position (heel-toe) before settling into the Riding Horse stance.

Posture movement:
As the front foot turns, the hands press down in front of the body (to the South) and then open up and out to the sides (initially palms down). The hands come above shoulder height and cross in front of the body above head height (palms facing away from each other). The hands come down in front of the body, 'framing the face', in their crossed position. They uncross in front of the abdomen and rise up and to the sides with palms down. The arms continue up to shoulder height with the right hand hanging down from the wrist so that the thumb contacts the fingers. The left hand's fingers point up so that the palm faces outwards to the side.

The Crane Exercises its Wings.
Move #13.

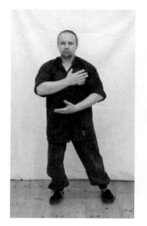 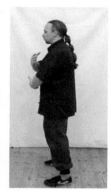

Stance: Right Leopard
Facing: South

<u>Stance movement:</u>

The weight shifts onto the right leg to come into Leopard stance.

<u>Posture movement:</u>

Hands return down and inwards with palms facing downwards. The hands then come in front of the body with the right hand coming up to position in front of the left shoulder with the palm facing inwards. The left hand comes into position, palm upwards, underneath the right elbow.

The Crane Exercises its Wings.
Move #14.

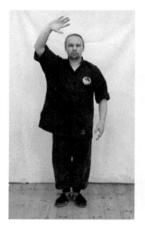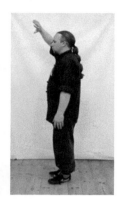

Stance: Eagle
Facing: South

Stance movement:

Draw the left leg in to place the heel next to the right heel, settling the weight into the left foot heel-toe. Then correct the right foot on the heel to point the toes out on the angle for Eagle stance.

Posture movement:

The right hand comes down in front of the body before rising up and out to the side. As the arm comes past shoulder height and the elbow starts to bend the palm turns to the front, the arm continues the circle to end in a 'salute' position at forehead level. The left hand comes down and to the side to finish in a relaxed position by the left hip.

Timing

Ensure that the stance movement and the hands are timed so that they all finish at the same time.

The Crane Exercises its Wings.
Move #15.

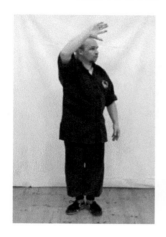 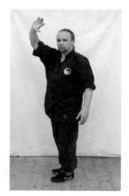

Stance: Eagle
Facing: South

Stance movement:

Throughout this move, maintain the Eagle stance.

Posture movement:

The upper body turns from the waist to face towards the East – maintain the stance with hips facing the front.

The Crane Exercises its Wings.
Move #16.

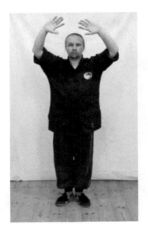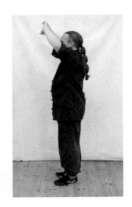

Stance: Eagle
Facing: South

<u>Stance movement:</u>

As with the previous move, maintain the Eagle stance during this movement.

<u>Posture movement:</u>

The upper body comes back into line with the hips (so facing back to the South). As it does this the left hand comes up and to the side as the right hand did in move #14 to finish in a 'double salute' position.

The Crane Exercises its Wings.
Move #17.

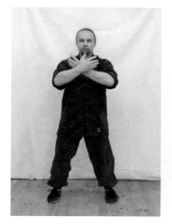 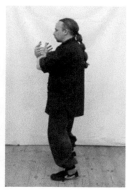

Stance: Riding Horse
Facing: South

<u>Stance movement:</u>

Move the weight onto the right foot, freeing the left foot and then move the left foot out to the side into position for the Riding Horse. Balance the weight across and slightly onto the left foot to allow you to correct the right foot (heel-toe!) before settling the weight into the Riding Horse stance.

<u>Posture movement:</u>

The arms separate out and to the sides coming down on their own respective sides of the body (palms downwards). As the hands reach the bottom part of their movement they continue in and across the body, coming up in a crossed position with the palms facing in towards the body until they are in front of the shoulders – often described as 'cupping the face'. Ensure that the wrists do not touch each other.

Drive the Tiger Away.
Move #18.

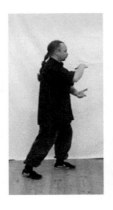 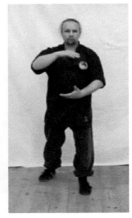

Stance: Left Dragon
Facing: South

<u>Stance movement:</u>

Shift the weight out of the left leg and onto the right, then step the left foot forwards into position for the Dragon stance (heel-toe, toes pointing forwards). Bring the weight forwards and into the Dragon stance correcting the right foot as you settle into the stance.

<u>Posture movement:</u>

Both hands lower down and towards their respective sides of the body with palms up until fingers are pointing forwards in front of the outside of the hips. Then imagine a large ball resting on both hands, rotate the ball so that the right hand comes on top of the 'ball' and the left hand underneath. Finishing with the right hand palm down at chest height facing towards the palm of the left hand which is palm up at Tantien height. The fingertips of both hands are pointing across the body.

Drive the Tiger Away.
Move #19.

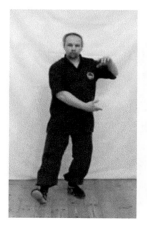 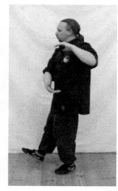

Stance: Right Monkey
Facing: South

Stance movement:

Draw the weight back from the Dragon stance into a left Duck stance. Then step the left foot back and continue to move the weight backwards to come into a right Duck stance before lifting the front toes to come into a Monkey stance.

Posture movement:

As you start to draw the weight back the hands start to rotate the 'ball' so that the left hand comes on top as you reach the left Duck stance. As the left foot steps back to come into the right Monkey, turn the upper body to the left to bring the 'ball' to the left side of the body. The head continues looking to the front (South).

Drive the Tiger Away.
Move #20.

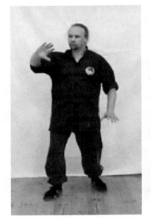 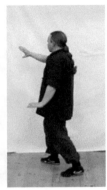

Stance: Right Dragon
Facing: South West

<u>Stance movement:</u>

Step the right foot so that it comes into position for the Dragon stance with the toes pointing to the South West. Bring the weight forward into Dragon stance.

<u>Posture movement:</u>

The left hand pushes down towards the right hand, giving a feeling of 'squeezing' the ball and pushing the right hand up and forwards to in front of the shoulder. As the hand comes forwards allow the hand to turn to palm facing away from the body. The left hand continues to press down to finish beside the left hip with the palm down.

Grasp the Bird's Tail.
Move #21.

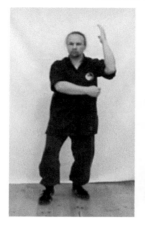 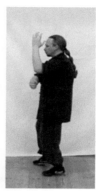

Stance: Right Cat
Facing: South

Stance movement:

The weight shifts backwards onto the back foot and the front foot then draws in before lifting the heel to come into the Cat stance.

Posture movement:

The right hand rolls forwards and over to form a loose fist with the thumb edge upwards. The right arm then circles in to bring the fist in towards the left side of the body just above hip height. The left hand circles in and upwards to finish at head height with the palm facing across the body and positioned just to the left of the head.

Grasp the Bird's Tail.
Move #22.

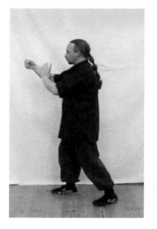 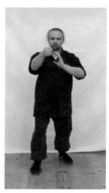

Stance: Right Dragon
Facing: West

Stance movement:

Stepping the right foot (heel-toe) to the right and then shifting the weight into it, come into a Dragon stance facing to the West. Correct the left foot as you settle into the stance – so as the hips come into alignment.

Posture movement:

The right hand, still in a loose fist, comes up and around to the right to around head height (think as if striking with the back of the fist). The left hand follows, to finish with the palm facing towards the mid-point of the right forearm, as if squeezing and pushing the right arm around.

Brush Knee and Sidestep.
Move #23.

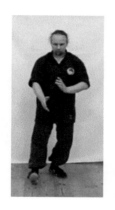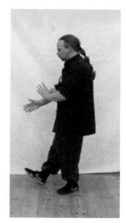

Stance: Right Monkey
Facing: West

Stance movement:

Draw the weight back on to the left foot and then lift the toes of the right foot to come into Monkey stance.

Posture movement:

The right hand opens from the fist to an open palm facing upwards. The hand then rolls outwards to the right and back over to palm downwards - so as if rolling around a ball that was held on the upturned palm. The hand continues to trace an 'S' shape by rolling inwards and up to palm upwards again above the point where the hand started. The hand then continues to turn to thumb edge upwards and, as the weight transfers back towards the Monkey stance, the hand 'cuts' downward with the little finger edge.

As you settle into the Monkey stance the upper body is inclined forwards a little to a point at which the head is looking towards a point on the floor around six feet in front of you.

Brush Knee and Sidestep.
Move #24.

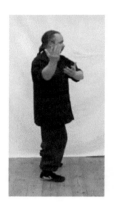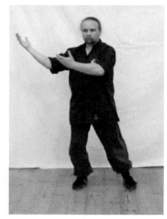

Stance: Right Leopard
Facing: South

Stance movement:

The front foot turns 90° on the heel so that the toes are pointing towards the South. The weight then shifts onto the right foot as the hips turn to also face South. Settle the weight onto the right leg and correct the left foot to come into a Leopard stance.

Posture movement:

The right hand circles in towards the body and then up inside the left arm to then 'roll over' the top of the left arm with the palm up. The left arm also rolls, initially forwards and down before coming to palm up. The arms then 'sweep' forwards and out to the right side of the body to finish with the right arm extended to the right, palm up, and the left hand in front of the right shoulder, palm up. As the arms sweep to the right, the head also looks to the right, before returning to a neutral position at the end of the move.

Repulse the Monkey.
Move #25.

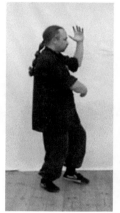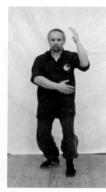

Stance: Left Cat
Facing: East

Stance movement:

Shift the weight onto the left leg and correct the right foot around 45° to the left. Transfer the weight back on to the right leg as you turn to face East. Draw the left leg in and then raise the heel to come in to a Cat stance.

Posture movement:

The right hand sweeps around in a circle with the palm facing in the direction of movement to finish with the palm facing in towards the waist on the left side of the body. The left forearm also sweeps around to come into a vertical position with the little finger edge forwards (hand around face height so the elbow is below shoulder height).

Timing

Hands and stance finish at the same time. The left foot should draw in to the Cat stance as the right hand draws in towards the waist.

Repulse the Monkey.
Move #26.

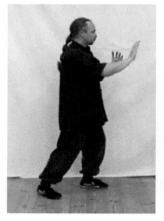 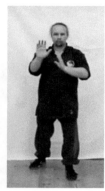

Stance: Left Dragon
Facing: East

Stance movement:

Step the left foot forwards and then transfer the weight into the Dragon stance.

Posture movement:

Turn the right hand to palm upwards and then draw it across the front of the body at waist height before raising to shoulder height so that both palms are facing each other as if holding a 'ball'. As the right hand moves across the body, there should be a turn of the upper body approximately 45° to the right. The right hand then 'pushes' with the palm forwards (to the East) to finish extended, in front of the right shoulder. The left hand lowers slightly to finish at chest height, just on the left side of the centre line.

Timing

The turn of the upper body coincides with the step of the left foot forwards and then the 'push' of the right hand coincides with the weight transfer into Dragon.

The Stork is Aroused.
Move #27.

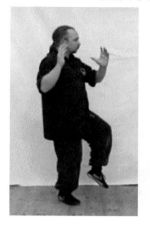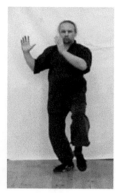

Stance: Left Crane
Facing: East

Stance movement:

Draw the weight back onto the right leg and then raise the left knee to come into a Crane stance with the lower leg hanging down from the knee, remembering to 'step' heel-toe with the left foot as you come into the stance.

Posture movement:

Bring the right hand down and back, maintaining the extension of the arm. The left hand follows the line of the right forearm (as if 'stroking' down the length of the right arm) to come into position as if holding a 'ball' as the hands both come to around waist height. The 'ball' is then circled slightly to the right side of the body, before continuing the circle to come into position where the 'ball' is held in front of the chest with fingers pointing upwards. The upper body is turned around 45° to the right so that it appears that the 'ball' is being held to the right side of the body.

The Stork is Aroused.
Move #28.

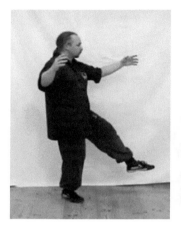 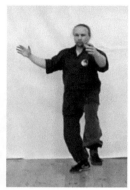

Stance: Left Dog
Facing: East

Stance movement:

Extend the left foot forwards into a Dog stance, remembering to 'step' heel-toe and not to over-straighten the leg or raise the leg too high.

Posture movement:

Expand the 'ball', keeping the palms of the hands facing each other. Start bringing the upper body back towards 'straight', so at the end of the move the upper body is still turned approximately 30° to the right.

The Stork is Aroused.
Move #29.

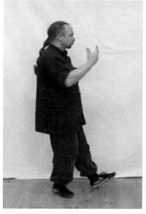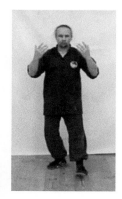

Stance: Left Monkey
Facing: East

<u>Stance movement:</u>

Lower the left leg to bring the heel onto the floor into a Monkey stance, before connecting the 'Bubbling Spring' point on the sole of the foot to the floor by lowering the foot into a Duck stance. Then, lift the toes of the left foot again to return to the Monkey stance. Ensure the weight remains on the back foot throughout the movement.

<u>Posture movement:</u>

Bring the upper body back into alignment with the hips, bringing the 'ball' in front of the shoulders. Lower the 'ball' in front of the body and then turn the palms in to face towards the body before they circle up to fingers pointing up, palms in, in front of the shoulders (similar to the first part of move #8 but do not extend the hands forwards).

<u>Timing</u>

The left leg lowers as the 'ball' is lowered in front of the body.

The Stork is Aroused.
Move #30.

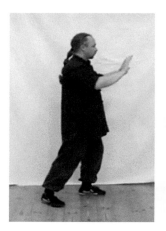 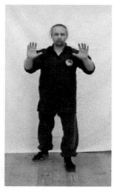

Stance: Left Dragon
Facing: East

<u>Stance movement:</u>
 The left foot steps forwards, heel-toe, before the weight is transferred forwards into Dragon stance.

<u>Posture movement:</u>
 Both hands turn inwards and then to palms forwards (as if circling around two 'balls'). The hands then extend forwards in a 'push' type movement similar to move #10.

The Double Whip.
Move #31.

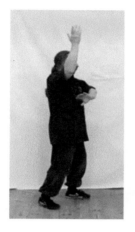 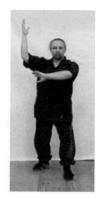

Stance: Left Snake
Facing: East

Stance movement:

The weight draws back into a Duck stance before moving forwards again into the Snake stance – make sure you do not come too far forwards and end in a Dragon.

Posture movement:

Both arms roll downwards and to the right side of the body. They then continue the same circle with the right arm staying extended and finishing with the right hand directed upwards (palm facing to the left). The circle of the left arm contracts to bring the left hand into position where it is 'guarding' the right armpit with the palm facing outwards.

Timing

The arms come downwards as the weight shifts back to Duck stance and then circle upwards as the weight comes into the Snake stance.

The Double Whip.
Move #32.

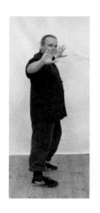 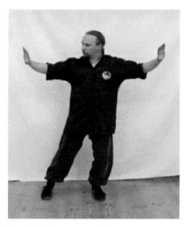

Stance: Left Leopard
Facing: South

Stance movement:

The weight rocks back onto the right leg and the left foot hooks 90° to the right (toes pointing towards South). Bring the weight onto the left leg and correct the right foot to come into a Leopard stance facing South with the weight on the left leg.

Posture movement:

The hands continue to move in the same circle as in the previous move and then split away from each other to come up and away from the body. The hands finish extended outwards at shoulder height with the palms facing away from the body. The head turns to look towards the right hand.

Timing

The head turns as the arms come up and outwards.

The Cobra Unwinds.
Move #33.

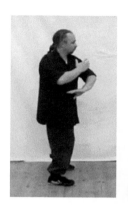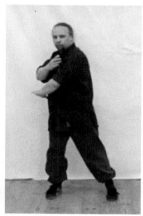

Stance: Right Leopard
Facing: South

Stance movement:

Transfer the weight over onto the right leg into a Right Leopard stance.

Posture movement:

Both arms come down and inwards. The right arm comes in and across the body so that the palm is facing in towards the left shoulder. The left hand finishes underneath the right elbow, with palm facing downwards.

The Cobra Unwinds.
Move #34.

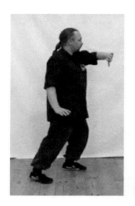 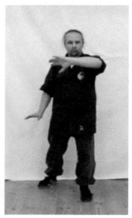

Stance: Left Dragon
Facing: South

Stance movement:

Step the left foot forwards and transfer the weight into Dragon stance, correcting the back foot out onto the angle.

Posture movement:

The left arm comes up and forwards in front of the body to finish with the left palm angled at roughly a 45° angle forwards and down – the arm is not extended too far forwards, think as if you are pushing away with the forearm, not the hand. The right hand moves down and back across the body to finish, palm down, beside the right hip. Keep the elbow relaxed and ensure that it is not pulled in tight to the body.

The Cobra Unwinds.
Move #35.

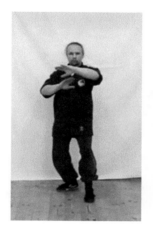 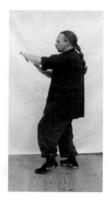

Stance: Left Cat
Facing: South

<u>Stance movement:</u>

Transfer the weight back onto the right leg and then draw the left leg, raising the heel to come into Cat stance.

<u>Posture movement:</u>

Keeping the palm facing downwards, the right hand comes up and outwards to circle back in towards the body, over the top of the left arm. Finish with the fingers of the right arm pointing towards the mid-point of the left forearm (making a capital letter 'T' shape with the arms).

The Cobra Unwinds.
Move #36.

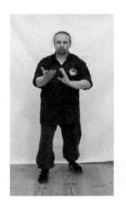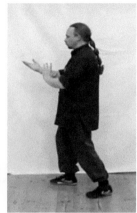

Stance: Right Dragon
Facing: West

Stance movement:

    Drop the heel of the left foot and then lift the toes before correcting it 45° to the right. Then, transfer the weight onto the left leg and step the right foot to the right into position for the Dragon stance. Transfer the weight into a Right Dragon stance.

Posture movement:

    The right hand 'pats' down towards the left knee and then 'scoops' upwards to come palm up in front of the body. The right hand then comes across the front of the body with the palm up to finish to the right-hand side of the body. The left hand 'squeezes' across as if pushing the right forearm into position, finishing just on the left side of the centre line.

Timing

    Drop the toes of the left foot as the right hand pats down and then lift the toes to correct the foot as the hand 'scoops' up.

The Wild Dog Retaliates.
Move #37.

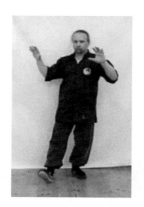 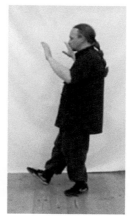

Stance: Right Monkey
Facing: West

Stance movement:

Draw the weight back onto the left leg and draw the right foot back in a short distance. After drawing the foot in, lift the toes of the right foot into Monkey stance.

Posture movement:

Both hands open outwards and come to palms up, they then continue to circle up and out until they are palms forwards at shoulder height.

The Wild Dog Retaliates.
Move #38.

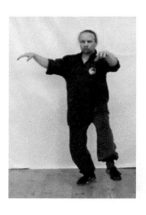 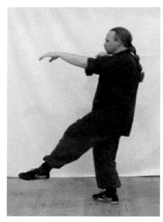

Stance: Left Dog
Facing: West

Stance movement:

Place the right foot down with the toes pointing out approximately 45° to the right. Transfer the weight onto the right leg and then bring the left leg through and up into Dog stance – keep the leg 'straight' as it comes up.

Posture movement:

Both hands press down and inwards before rising back up and out to shoulder height with the palms down (hands finish slightly wider than shoulder width apart).

Timing

Place the right foot down as the hands press down, and lift the left leg as the hands come up.

The Wild Dog Retaliates.
Move #39.

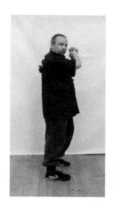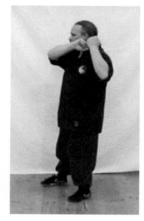

Stance: Left Leopard
Facing: South-West

Stance movement:

The left leg continues outward to the left, then place the left foot down to your left with the toes pointing out on a 45° angle. Transfer the weight onto your left leg and then correct the right foot to come into a Leopard stance.

Posture movement:

The arms bend at the elbows as the right hand comes across to position itself in a loose fist with the back of the hand beside the left ear (thumb edge downwards). The left hand also comes into a soft fist with the palm facing the palm of the right hand (little finger edge pointing forwards). The head is directed towards the West, looking over the right elbow.

The Wild Dog Retaliates.
Move #40.

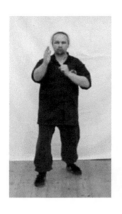 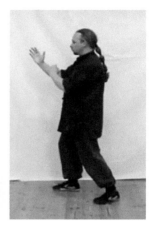

Stance: Right Dragon
Facing: West

Stance movement:

Step the right foot to come into a Dragon stance facing West. Note that you should have moved about a half step to the left since the Dragon stance in move #36.

Posture movement:

The right hand opens so that the palm is facing in towards the left ear. Bring the right hand around the back of the head so that the palm faces in towards the back of the neck and then the right ear. The right hand then 'cuts' down to shoulder height, advanced in front of the right shoulder. The left hand moves down and across until it is in front of the chest, slightly to the left of the centre line (still in a fist).

The Tail of the Peacock.
Move #41.

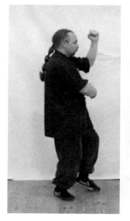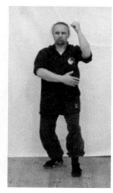

Stance: Left Cat
Facing: East

Stance movement:

Shift the weight back onto the left leg and then correct the right foot around so that the toes are pointing towards the South-East. Bring the weight back onto the right foot as the body turns to face East drawing the left foot back and in to come into Cat stance.

Posture movement:

The right hand sweeps around, down and in, to 'wrap' around the waist, finishing with the palm facing the waist on the left side of the centre line. The left hand (still in a fist) comes up and out to finish with the forearm pointing upwards in front of the left shoulder, with the little finger edge pointing forwards and the hand at head height.

Timing

Draw the left foot in as the right hand sweeps in towards the waist.

The Tail of the Peacock.
Move #42.

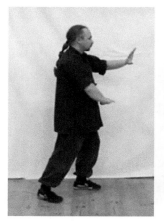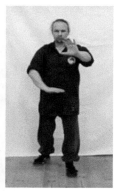

Stance: Left Dragon
Facing: East

Stance movement:

Step the left foot forwards and then bring the weight through into the Dragon stance.

Posture movement:

Open the left hand, bring the right hand across the body at waist height (palm up) and then up to make a 'ball' with the palms facing each other and fingers pointing up (hands at shoulder height). The right hand then continues to roll over to palm down and presses down in front of the centre line. The left hand turns to push forwards with the palm, until extended in front of the left shoulder.

Timing

Bring the weight forwards into the Dragon as the left hand pushes forwards.

The Tail of the Peacock.
Move #43.

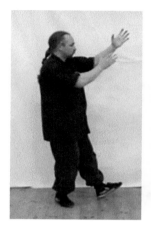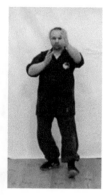

Stance: Left Monkey
Facing: East

Stance movement:

Transfer the weight back onto the right leg, draw the left leg back inwards a short distance and then lift the toes of the left foot into Monkey stance.

Posture movement:

Both hands circle forwards and upwards with the palms turning so that thumb edges are upwards and fingers forwards. The arms continue to circle over and back in to come into a high 'en-garde' position.

The Tail of the Peacock.
Move #44.

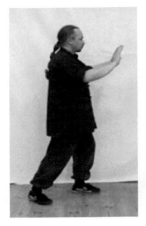 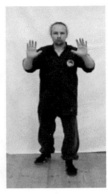

Stance: Left Dragon
Facing: East

Stance movement:

Step the left foot forwards and bring the weight through into Dragon stance.

Posture movement:

The hands continue to circle in and down and then split to turn around two 'balls' in front of the shoulders before pushing forwards with the palms (similar to move #10).

Timing

Bring the weight forwards into Dragon as the palms press forwards.

Brush Knee and Sidestep.
Move #45.

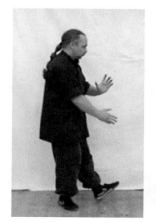 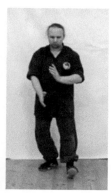

Stance: Left Monkey
Facing: East

Stance movement:

    Bring the weight back onto the right leg, drawing the left foot in before lifting the toes into Monkey stance.

Posture movement:

    The right hand makes a similar movement to move #23, this time opening to palm up and rolling over to the top of a 'ball' and then cutting down through the centre of the ball. The upper body bends forwards slightly from the waist as the hand 'cuts' down so that you finish with your head looking to the floor approximately 6 feet in front of you. The left hand turns inwards to come into position, fingers pointing up, little finger edge forwards, just on the left side of the centre line at mid-chest height.

Timing

    Ensure the weight is back and the toes are lifted before leaning forwards.

Brush Knee and Sidestep.
Move #46.

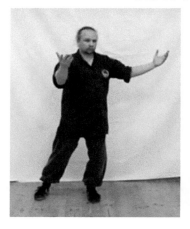 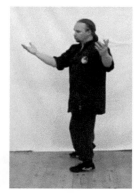

Stance: Left Leopard
Facing: South

Stance movement:

The left foot hooks 90° to the right, stepping slightly forward so the toes are pointing South. Shift the weight onto the left leg and correct the right foot into Leopard stance.

Posture movement:

The right hand rolls in and up (on the inside of the left arm) as the left arm rolls out and down – this brings the right hand over the top of the left forearm with both palms up. The arms then open outwards and upwards to finish palms up at shoulder height with the arms extended. The upper body is turned slightly to the left so that the right arm extends to the front and the left arm out to the left side.

Timing

The arms 'fold' as the foot hooks and then the arms sweep out as you come into the Leopard stance.

The Edge of the Cyclone.
Move #47.

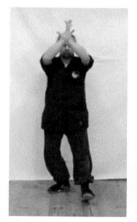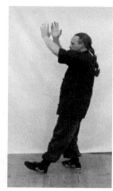

Stance: Left Monkey
Facing: South

Stance movement:

Step the right foot backwards and bring the weight back onto the right leg. Lift the toes of the left foot to come into Monkey stance.

Posture movement:

The arms continue up and outward, then cross (left arm around right) above head height. Finishing with palms facing outwards (little finger edges facing forwards).

The Edge of the Cyclone.
Move #48.

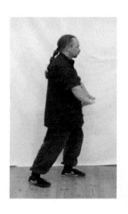 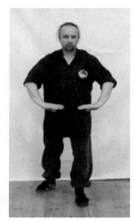

Stance: Right Dragon
Facing: South

Stance movement:

Correct the toes of the left foot outwards 45° and then step the right foot through, following with the weight to come into Right Dragon.

Posture movement:

The arms come down in front of the body, uncrossing as they reach Tantien height. They continue to circle out from the body and up to come just over shoulder height with the palms down (fingertips pointing at fingertips). The hands then press down in front of the body, either side of the centre line to Tantien level. At the end of the move the upper body turns slightly to the right so that if you were to look down you would see the right thigh between the hands.

Timing

Step the foot as the arms come up, transferring the weight into Dragon as the hands press down.

The Edge of the Cyclone.
Move #49.

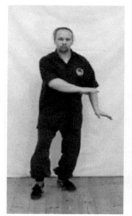 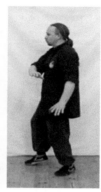

Stance: Right Cat
Facing: South

Stance movement:

Transfer the weight back onto the left leg and then draw in the right foot, lifting the heel into Cat stance.

Posture movement:

The right hand circles forward and to the left, staying palm down and at Tantien height. The left hand turns to point the fingers to the left, away from the body, still palm down.

The Edge of the Cyclone.
Move #50.

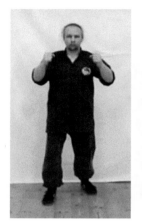 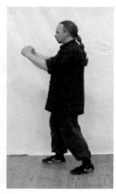

Stance: Right Dragon
Facing: South

Stance movement:

Step the right foot forwards and then transition the weight forwards into Dragon stance.

Posture movement:

The hands form into loose fists and come to in front of the body (either side of the centre line at Tantien height). The arms then drift forwards and upwards to finish at shoulder height in soft fists with the thumb edge pointing upwards.

Gather Earth's Energy.
Closing.

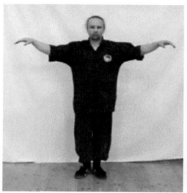 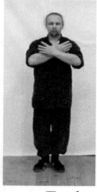 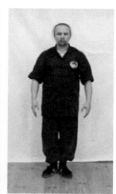

Stance: Eagle
Facing: South

Stance movement:

Draw the right foot back and into Eagle stance.

Posture movement:

Both hands open and circle down towards a 'neutral' position hanging by the sides. Both hands move up and outwards to shoulder height, palms down out to the sides (image 1). Roll the hands back down and inwards towards the body and then up in front of the body with the right hand crossed over the left, palms facing in towards the body. The hands come up until they are facing in towards the shoulders (image 2) and then roll back down in front of the body, slowly uncrossing so that when they reach Tantien height the right hand palm is facing the back of the left hand and the left palm is facing the Tantien. The hands then continue to uncross and finish hanging in the neutral position by the sides (image 3).

Section 3a.

Refinements of the
Taiji Short Form.

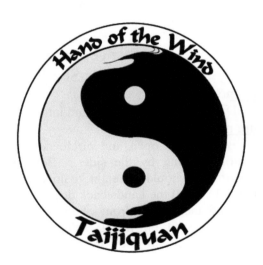

Refinements of the Movements of the Taiji Short Form.

As you train within a Taijiquan system, your body gradually softens and relaxes and so it is important that you always revisit all of the moves of your Form. Even after you have been training for many years, there will still be things that you need to improve and refine in every movement.

The following section of this book is intended for more experienced students, who have learnt the full Short Form and are looking for ways to get more out of their Taiji practice. The following notes are simply intended to give ideas and directions for students to explore, in order to refine their Taiji Form movements. The comments and ideas are not intended to tell you how to do the movements, they are intended to make you think about and engage with the movements of <u>your</u> Form.

Taiji Short Form Refinements.

1   Ensure the timing of posture and stance coincide by ensuring that the fingers are pointing forwards at the point when the heels touch. Settle the weight into both feet as the hands come in towards the centre.
There should be a feeling of opening of the upper back between the shoulder blades and a collapsing of the chest as we come into position at the end of the move.

2   Ensure that the shoulders do not lift as the arms rise. Also, be aware that the amount of bend at the elbow should not change as the arms lift, think of a simple rotation of the shoulder.
Do not try to look up to such an extent that it introduces tension to the back of the neck. Consider how the chest lifts to 'roll' the head back instead.

3   As in move #2 the arms maintain their shape as they lower, again using a relaxed rotation of the shoulders.
Consider how an inward movement of the elbows can initiate the rotation of the hands from palm down to palm up.

4 Consider how collapsing the chest allows the right hand to move over the top of the left hand.

5 As the hands come around the ball be aware of the opening of the chest.
In the 'en-garde' position there should be a feeling of the palms slightly pushing in towards the plane of the centre line of the body - this is initiated from the centre of the body, do not press in with the hands or elbows.

6 Consider similarities with move #4.
Movement of the hands should come from the centre – think about how the waist, shoulders and chest interact.

7 Consider similarities to move #5, the differences come towards the end of the move. How does the hip draw the right hand into position?
Don't drop the chin to look down, maintain the neck alignment and use the back.
The left hand should be fractionally to its own side of the centre line and the right should line up with the outside of the hip.

8 Ensure the movement of the hands is from the centre of the body and that the wrists stay relaxed.
The hands do not move 'forward' very far in reality, the movement of the stance makes it look like a bigger movement than it is.

9 As in move #8 keep the hand movement small and driven by the body.
The hand movements of move #10 are already beginning as you settle into the Monkey stance – remember the numbers are a guide!

10 As in moves #8 and #9 the actual distance moved by the hands relative to the body is actually very small.
Focus on the movement of the body and the hands will take care of themselves!

11 As with all the movements of 'Fair Lady Weaving' the hands move a small distance relative to the body. Be aware of the position of the elbows and keeping the wrists relaxed - don't allow the elbows to be 'squeezed' in towards each other in front of the body.

12
As the hands rise and fall be aware of the lift of the body in the stance through high and low Riding Horse stances.
Ensure that the hands are not stretched too far out to the sides at the end of the move – there should be a feeling of the arms forming part of a circle.

13
Consider how a collapsing of the chest can bring the hands into position without tightening the upper arms in too close to the body and thus causing tension.

14
It is the timing of this move that causes most people problems – ensure all aspects of the movement are driven from the Tantien.
At the end of the move the fingertips of the right hand are across the centre line – but not Laogong point.

15
Think about the upward circle of the right arm in the previous move and how that is continued through the body during the turn.
At the end of the move the fingertips of the right hand should no longer be across the centerline of the forehead.

Be aware of any build-up of tension in the shoulders or back during these moves – keep them relaxed by moving from the centre.

16 Although the stance stays in Eagle throughout these movements ensure the stance isn't rigid – again, stay relaxed.

Consider how the initial movement of the right arm is tied to the movement of the left leg.

17 In order to bring the hands across the centre-line of the body allow the chest to 'collapse' rolling the shoulders forwards and expanding between the shoulder-blades.

As always, ensure the hand and stance movement are synchronized and finish together.

18 Consider how the elbows move as the arms complete the movement.

19 Be aware of the position of the hands when holding the 'ball', the bottom hand should be in front of the lower Tantien and the upper in front of the middle Tantien, Laogong points should be lined up with each other. Try collapsing the chest a bit to bring the hands into position.
When you bring the 'ball' to the side be aware that this is a turn of the upper body and not a movement of the hands to the side.

20 If the Dragon stance is properly aligned there should be little need to correct the left foot.
At the end of the move the left hand should be in a relaxed position – consider the position of the elbow, being aware of critical distance.

21 Even though this is considered to be facing South the stance is still facing slightly West of South (so a little to the left), the upper body is turned slightly from the waist in relation to the stance so the shoulders are square to the South.

22 As the right fist comes to head height make sure that the arm is not lifted from the shoulder – think about the alignment and opening of the chest as a means to lift the arm instead.

23 Consider how the movement of the hand is generated from the Tantien – focus on the back of the left hip. To remember the hand movement, the martial aspect of throat-eyes-forehead can sometimes be useful!

24 As the right foot and lower leg is pushing forwards the arms are sweeping to the rear – be aware of the 'scissoring' nature of the movement. As the arms sweep to the right the upper body turns to the right (creating the 'look' to the left) and then at the end of the move straighten the body somewhat which initiates the start of move #25

25 Pay particular attention to the feeling of the right hand 'drawing in' the left foot. Consider the timing of the turn of the waist as you come around into the Cat stance.

26 Think about how the turn of the upper body and the timing of the ward off work with the step of the foot forwards – how is the hip orientated?

27 Be aware of the circle the hands make as it rolls to the side of the body – there is almost a feeling of the hands going behind the body, although this is created by the turn of the waist.

28 This is another movement which provides an illusory sense of the arms being held out to the front and the side, whereas they are actually held in a symmetrical position and it is the turn of the waist that makes it look as if the left hand is extended forwards.

29 Consider the circle that the arms move in during the whole movement – there should not be a feeling of a change of direction at the bottom of the hands movement.

30 Be aware of how the circular movement of the arms at the end of the last move is transformed by the turn of the hands, enabling the forward 'push' to go 'under the ball'.

31 Consider the angle of the upper body throughout the arm movements. Remember that the left forearm is advanced in order to provide the feeling of a 'ward-off' or 'Peng'.

32 Consider the similarities between the hook of the foot and the arm movements in this move with each of the 'Brush Knee and Sidestep' sequences.

33 This is another movement where the angle of the upper body, created by the turning of the waist is critical. Also, be aware of the 'collapsing' of the chest which allows the hands to cross over the centre-line of the body.

34 Be aware of the left forearm, keep your intent in the feeling of the push or 'ward-off' focused along the edge of the bone in the forearm.

35 The movement of the body should create a circle with the left arm and the right hand, so be aware of the isolation of the right shoulder joint.

36 In order to create the feeling of the 'squeeze' with the left hand, consider the collapse of the chest. Be aware of the final position of the right hand to ensure that it is not too high.

37 This is a movement where you can really focus on the expansion of the chest and how it creates the correct arm movement.

38 As the leg comes up into Dog stance, remember that it makes an arc that comes inwards and then outwards. In a martial sense, think as if kicking with the little toe edge of the foot as it swings outwards.

39 The left leg should continue the outward circle from the previous movement and then be aware of where you place the foot down. This is the point at which you ensure that you move to your left during this sequence.

40 Think about the isolation and relaxation of the right shoulder as the right hand passes the back of the head – ensure that the shoulder does not lift too high during the movement.

41 Consider how, in martial application, the turn and the arm movements provide a guard against both low and high attacks coming from an attacker positioned behind you. Be aware of how the concept of the Taiji Form only going to the point of contact affects how this movement differs from the application.

42 The martial application (inward arm ward off with left arm, followed by inward arm movement with right arm before the press down and strike) is particularly useful to aid in the visualization of this movement. Consider the timing of the step and the movements of the arms.

43 Be aware of the difference in feeling of the 'rolling over' backward movement in this move compared to other movements in the Form where we move back from Dragon to Monkey.

44 As with other movements which feature the hands turning as if 'around two balls', be aware of the directions of the circles that the hand movements make.

45 Consider the timing of the movements of both arms – as the right hand opens to palm up, what happens through the body? What effect does this have on the timing of the movement of the left hand?

46 Consider the similarity of arm position at the end of this move and move #28 – again be aware of the turn of the upper body and its effect on the arm position.

47 Be conscious of the angle of the body during the step and how this enables the left arm to cross in front of the right. Again, it is the collapse of the chest that allows the arms to cross the centre-line.

48 As you bring the weight forwards, be aware of focusing your intent into the front of the right shoulder and upper arm – in martial application this would be one of the points of contact with the opponent.

49 Another movement where the arms appear to be on one side of the body – consider the turn from the waist and how it enables you to avoid being 'double-weighted' and off-balance.

50 Be aware of the uncoiling of the waist and how it coincides with the closing of the fists – pay particular attention to the transition from horizontal circle to vertical.
Remember to keep relaxed – especially if you are completing the short Form and are feeling jubilant!

Section 4.

Taiji Feishou Form.

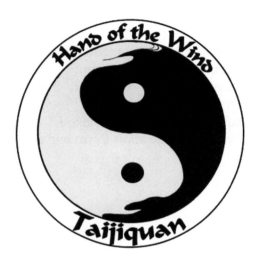

Taiji Feishou Form

The Feishou Form is often described as a 'Fast Form' and sometimes as the 'Taiji dance'. Both of these can give a false impression of the Feishou to students – there is just as much detail to consider as in the main Form and although it can feel more flowing, due to the nature of the movements, it should not be performed much faster than the Form.

The Feishou also incorporates many excellent martial applications and I consider it to be a vital area of study for students of the martial aspects of our style – when it is referred to as a 'dance' this can have the effect of putting some students off this Form. For these reasons, within our classes we refer to this as the Feishou Form.

This section describes the first thirty movements of the Feishou. As with section 3, the moves are broken up into stance, posture and timing notes. Images are provided from more than one viewpoint. Again, these notes provide compass directions for facing and, as with the Form notes, these are for reference only.

Feishou Form Quick Reference Table

Move	Stance	Facing
Start	Eagle	South
Prepare	Bear	"
1	Eagle	"
2	Right Dragon	West
3	Eagle	South
4	Left Dragon	East
5	Left Duck	"
6	Right Dragon	"
7	Left Leopard	South
8	Left Crane	East
9	Eagle	South
10	Right Leopard	"
11	Left Dragon	East
12	Right Dragon	West
13	Left Dragon	East
14	Left Duck	"
15	Left Crane	"
16	Left Leopard	South
17	Left Dragon	East
18	Left Cat	"
19	Left Dragon	"
20	Right Dragon	"
21	Right Chicken	"
22	Left Duck	West
23	Left Dog	"
24	Left Dragon	"
25	Left Dragon	"
26	Right Dragon	"
27	Left Dragon	"
28	Left Leopard	North
29	Right Dragon	East
30	Right Cat	"

Prepare.

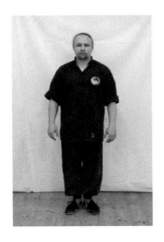 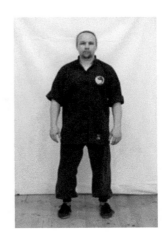

Stance: Bear
Facing: South

Stance movement:

As with the Form, in order to begin the Feishou we prepare by stepping from an Eagle stance into Bear stance. This is done by stepping the left foot to the left, placing the heel down and then the toes making sure that the foot is aligned to point forwards. The right foot is then corrected heel-toe to bring the feet into the correct parallel orientation for the Bear stance.

Posture movement:

Arms stay, hanging relaxed, by your sides.

Move #1.

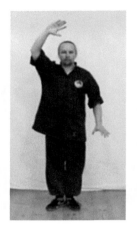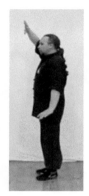

Stance: Eagle
Facing: South

Stance movement:

Similar to move #1 of the Form; correct the right foot and then draw the left foot back in to Eagle stance.

Posture movement:

The right hand comes up and away from the body in a large circle, continuing to come into a 'salute' position with the back of the hand facing the forehead. The left hand comes into an 'active' position with the palm facing the floor – ensuring that the elbow is not held tight into the body.

Move #2.

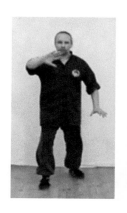 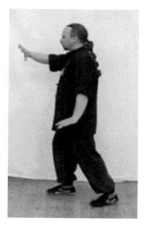

Stance: Right Dragon
Facing: West

<u>Stance movement:</u>

Similar to move #6 of the Form. The right foot swings around to the right and is placed down heel-toe. The weight then transfers onto the right foot and as the hips come into alignment for the Dragon stance correct the left foot heel-toe. Consider where you place the right foot to ensure you end in a good Dragon stance and not 'on line'.

<u>Posture movement:</u>

The right hand continues its circle to come down the front of the body, on the left side of the centre-line. The circle continues to swing the right hand up and forward to in front of the right shoulder. The left hand remains in an active position near the left hip.

Move #3.

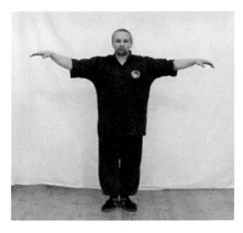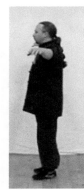

Stance: Eagle
Facing: South

Stance movement:

Spin towards the right (clockwise) on the right foot coming all the way around to face the South. The left foot lands in position with the heel touching the right heel to come into an Eagle stance.

Posture movement:

The left hand swings up and out from the body so that both arms are extended out to the sides during the spin, with the palms turned outwards (away from the body). At the end of the movement, both arms are still extended out to the sides at shoulder height with the palms down.

Timing:

As the left hand swings up and out, it lifts the left foot to initiate the spin.

Move #4.

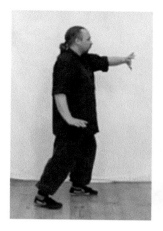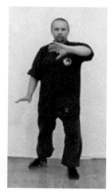

Stance: Left Dragon
Facing: East

<u>Stance movement:</u>

Similar to move #2, except this time step the left foot to the left to come into a Left Dragon facing towards the East.

<u>Posture movement:</u>

Both arms lift upwards and then circle down in front of the body so that the arms cross, left arm around the right. As the hands come down to hip height, the right hand remains in an active position beside the right hip. The left hand continues the circle to come up and to the front to finish in front of the left shoulder.

<u>Timing:</u>

The step to the left coincides with the left arm coming upwards and away from the body.

Move #5.

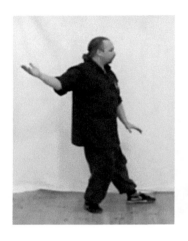 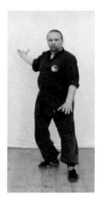

Stance: Left Duck
Facing: East

Stance movement:

    Shift the weight back onto the right leg, drawing the left foot in slightly to come into a Duck stance.

Posture movement:

    Both hands turn towards each other, as if holding a 'ball'. The right hand then splits off the ball to come up and out the side, passing just above shoulder height at the point when it is fully extended to the side. The right hand continues this circle to extend behind the body at shoulder height with the palm facing upwards. When the left hand splits off the ball it circles down in front of the body to finish in an active position in front of the left hip.

Move #6.

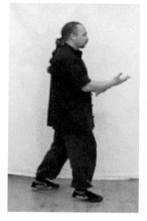 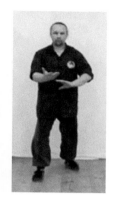

Stance: Right Dragon
Facing: East

<u>Stance movement:</u>

Correct the left foot out 45° to the left and then bring the weight forwards onto the left leg. Step the right foot through, placing the foot into position to be able to bring the weight onto the right leg and into a Dragon stance.

<u>Posture movement:</u>

The right hand circles to palm down and then returns back along the reverse of the course it followed in the previous move; just above shoulder height as it extends to the side and then rolling down to underneath the left hand. As the right hand passes underneath the left hand, it turns to palm up and then extends forwards from underneath the left hand to out in front of the body, followed by the left hand – similar to move #4 of the Taiji Form, but with the left hand palm down.

<u>Timing:</u>

Correct the left foot as the right hand turns palm down. Bring the weight into the left leg as the right hand comes 'down the slide' and step forward as the right hand comes out from under the left hand.

Move #7.

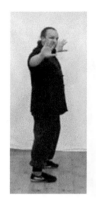 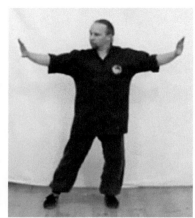

Stance: Left Leopard
Facing: South

Stance movement:
  Step the left foot through and hook it around so that the toes point 90° to the left. Bring the weight on to the left leg and then correct the right foot to come into the Leopard stance.

Posture movement:
  Bring the left hand up and over the right hand as if taking hold of a 'ball'. Then raise the ball in front of the body (palms facing each other) until the fingers are pointing upwards. The hands then 'drop' the ball and move down and outwards to come up and out to the sides (shoulder height with palms facing outwards).

Timing:
  Step the left foot through as the left hand comes over the right hand to form the 'ball'.

Move #8.

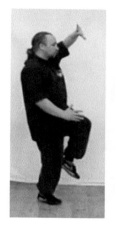 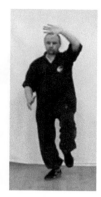

Stance: Left Crane
Facing: East

Stance movement:

Correct the right foot approximately 45° to the left and then transfer the weight onto the right leg. Turn the hips to the left and raise the left leg to come into Crane stance facing East. Remember that in the Feishou (unlike the Form) the raised foot is pulled back towards the standing leg.

Posture movement:

Both hands come down and inwards to in front of the hips. The left hand then drifts up and out, with the palm outwards and the little finger edge up to come into a 'salute' position. The right hand follows a circle to come to the left and then back in so that the palm is facing in towards the left thigh.

Timing:

The left leg lifts into Crane as the left hand comes up to the 'salute' position. The left foot pulls back in as the right hand circles in towards the body at the end of the movement.

Move #9.

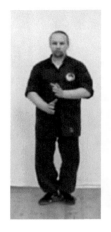 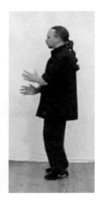

Stance: Eagle
Facing: South

<u>Stance movement:</u>

Correct the right foot as the weight is 'bounced' upwards and then lower the left leg to come into a deep Eagle stance (both knees more bent than usual).

<u>Posture movement:</u>

The left hand continues its upward movement and the shoulders turn to the right (to face South). The left hand follows the circle to come down in front of the body. When the left hand reaches the bottom of the circle, both hands move up and out to the sides and then down in front of the body following the centre-line. The right hand is below the left hand, with the fingers of both hands pointing to the front.

<u>Timing:</u>

Turn the upper body to face the front as the left hand comes down and then turn the hips as both hands rise and the weight is 'bounced' up out of the standing foot.

Move #10.

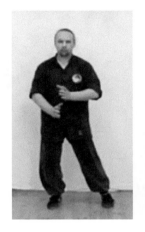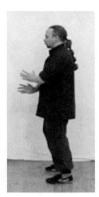

Stance: Right Leopard
Facing: South

Stance movement:

The left foot 'pushes' out to the left to come into a Leopard stance.

Posture movement:

The hands remain in position from the previous movement.

Move #11.

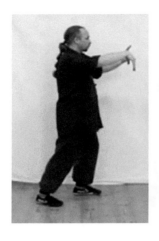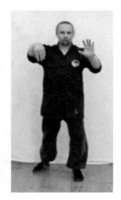

Stance: Left Dragon
Facing: East

Stance movement:

Step the left foot to the left, pointing the toes towards the East. Transfer the weight into the left leg and then correct the right foot into Dragon stance as the hips come around.

Posture movement:

Both hands drop and then drift up and forwards to an extended position in front of the shoulders. The left hand is fingers up, palm facing forwards and the right hand is fingers pointing downwards.

Move #12.

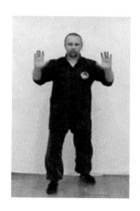 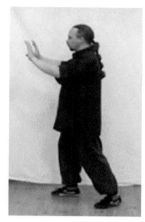

Stance: Right Dragon
Facing: West

Stance movement:

Draw the weight back onto the right leg, turn the front foot to bring the toes around approximately 135° to the right, the hips turn as the weight transitions onto the left leg. Step the right foot and then bring the weight forwards onto it to complete a 180° turn into a Right Dragon facing West.

Posture movement:

The right hand 'wipes' up and then down to match the left hand and then both hands drift downwards to around Tantien height before rising back up to shoulder height again with both hands having the palms facing forwards.

Timing:

As the body turns, the hands are at the bottom of their arc.

Move #13.

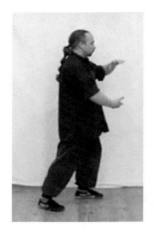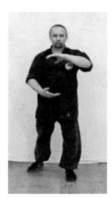

Stance: Left Dragon
Facing: East

Stance movement:

Transition the weight back onto the right leg and then turn the right foot inwards around 135°. Transfer the weight onto the right foot and step the left foot around before bringing the weight onto it into a Dragon stance, again having turned 180°.

Posture movement:

The hands roll in a clockwise circle to a position where they are holding a 'ball' with the left hand directly above the right hand. The body then turns whilst holding the 'ball'.

Timing:

Take hold of the 'ball' before turning, make sure you finish in Dragon and not Duck stance.

Move #14.

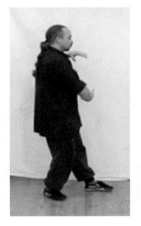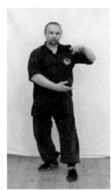

Stance: Left Duck
Facing: East

Stance movement:

Bring the weight back onto the right foot, drawing the left foot inwards a short distance to come into Duck stance.

Posture movement:

Still holding the 'ball' from the previous movement, turn the upper body from the waist to bring the ball to the left side of the body.

Move #15.

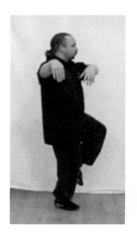 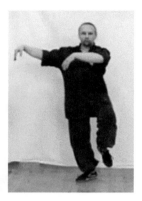

Stance: Left Crane
Facing: East

Stance movement:

Draw the left leg up off the floor into Crane stance, remembering to pull the heel in towards the body at the end of the movement.

Posture movement:

The right hand drifts across, in front of the body and then extends up and out to the side, with the fingertips pointing downwards (thumb edge forwards). The left hand drifts across the front of the chest in a circular movement to also finish with the fingertips pointing downwards

Move #16.

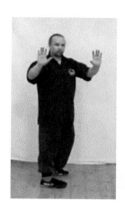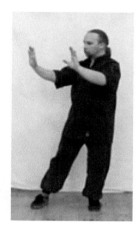

Stance: Left Leopard
Facing: South

Stance movement:

Place the left foot down, pointing the toes 90° to the right (facing South) and in line with the right foot. Transfer the weight onto the left leg and correct the right foot on the heel to come into a Leopard stance.

Posture movement:

Both hands roll over to push away from the body with the heels of the palms. As you settle into the stance, the upper body is turned 45° to the right.

Move #17.

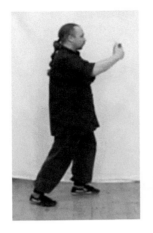 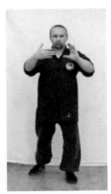

Stance: Left Dragon
Facing: East

Stance movement:

Correct the right foot 45° to the left and then transfer the weight onto the right leg. Step the left foot around to the left and then transition the weight onto the left leg to come into Dragon stance facing East.

Posture movement:

The right hand rolls to palm facing in towards the body with the thumb edge upwards. The left hand turns 45° to the right so that the fingertips of the right hand are directed towards the palm of the left hand. The hands remain in this posture as we turn into the Dragon stance.

Move #18.

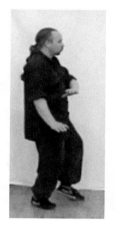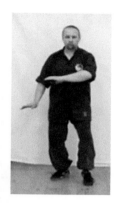

Stance: Left Cat
Facing: East

<u>Stance movement:</u>

Transfer the weight back onto the right leg and then draw the left foot in before lifting the left heel into Cat stance.

<u>Posture movement:</u>

The hands both circle to the left and then down in front of the body. The left hand finishes, palm down and fingertips pointing to the right, at elbow height. The right hand finishes, also palm down and fingertips pointing right, beside the right hip. The upper body is turned slightly to the right.

Move #19.

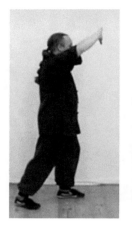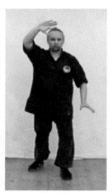

Stance: Left Dragon
Facing: East

<u>Stance movement:</u>

Step the left foot forward, heel-toe, before transferring the weight onto the left leg to come into Dragon stance.

<u>Posture movement:</u>

The right hand drifts up and forward to come into a 'salute' position – ensure the chest opens to lift the arm, rather than lifting the shoulder. The left hand turns across the front of the body to finish fingers pointing towards the left, palm down, beside the left hip.

Move #20.

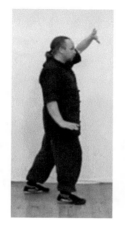 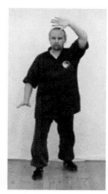

Stance: Right Dragon
Facing: East

Stance movement:

Step the right foot through in a 'long' ladder step to come into a right Dragon, correcting the left foot on the heel as the weight settles into the stance.

Posture movement:

Reverse the position of the hands, so that the left hand turns and drifts up the centre line to come into a 'salute' position. The right hand drifts down the centre line and then turns into position by the right hip. Again, be aware of the opening of the chest.

Move #21.

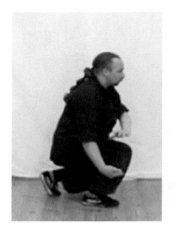 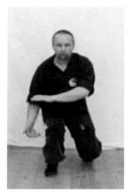

Stance: Right Chicken
Facing: East

<u>Stance movement:</u>

Raising the left heel off the floor, lower down into a Chicken stance (maintain 80% weight in the right leg – do not allow left knee to touch floor).

<u>Posture movement:</u>

The left hand rolls over and down the centre line as the body turns to the right. The right hand 'scoops' to come into position, palm up, under the left hand as if holding a 'ball'.

Move #22.

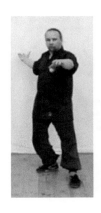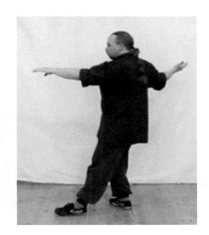

Stance: Left Duck
Facing: West

Stance movement:

Turn anti-clockwise 180°, allowing the left foot to swing a short distance to the left and pivoting on the right heel (keep weight on the right leg) to come into a left Duck stance.

Posture movement:

The hands split off the 'ball' so that the left hand comes up and forwards to finish, palm down, extended to the front at shoulder height. The right hand also splits up and out to finish at shoulder height, palm up, directed outwards to the rear of the body (be aware of the turn of the waist!).

Move #23.

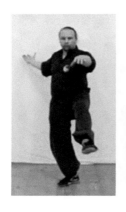 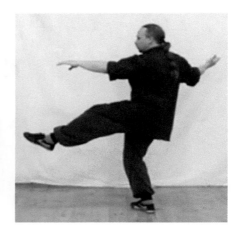

Stance: Left Dog
Facing: West

Stance movement:
 The left leg lifts off the floor to come into Dog stance.

Posture movement:
 The arms stay in the same position through this movement.

Move #24.

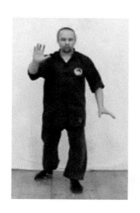 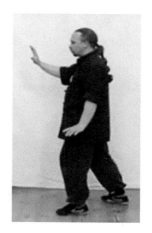

Stance: Left Dragon
Facing: West

Stance movement:

Place the left foot back down onto the floor and transition the weight into the left leg to come into Dragon stance.

Posture movement:

The right hand 'pushes' forwards, in an under-arm motion, to finish extended in front of the right shoulder. The left hand drifts down, to come into an 'active' position, palm down, beside the left hip.

Move #25.

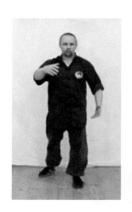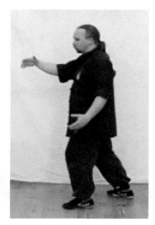

Stance: Left Dragon
Facing: West

Stance movement:

    Maintain the stance through this movement.

Posture movement:

    Roll both hands so that they come to holding a 'ball', palms facing each other. The right hand is still in front of the right shoulder and the left hand is still beside the left hip.

Move #26.

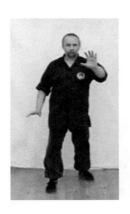 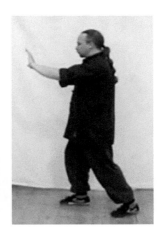

Stance: Right Dragon
Facing: West

Stance movement:

Step the right foot through in a 'long' ladder step to come into a right Dragon stance.

Posture movement:

The left hand 'pushes' forwards, in an over-arm motion, to finish extended in front of the right shoulder. The right hand drifts down, to come into an 'active' position, palm down, beside the left hip.

Move #27.

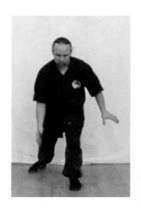 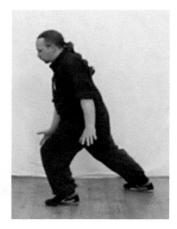

Stance: Left Dragon
Facing: West

Stance movement:

Once again, step the left foot through into a left Dragon stance in a 'long' ladder step.

Posture movement:

Roll through the body so that the left hand returns to an 'active' position beside the left hip. The right hand comes over shoulder height to 'cut' downwards. The body leans forwards from the waist to bring the right hand into a position where the palm is facing in towards the left knee. It is important to ensure that you remain in a correct Dragon stance, even when the body is leaning.

Move #28.

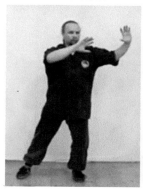 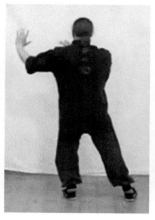 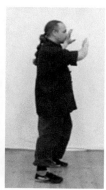

Stance: Left Leopard
Facing: North

<u>Stance movement:</u>

Briefly, transition the weight into the right leg to allow you to hook the left foot 90° to the right and into line with the right foot. Transfer the weight back onto the left leg and correct the right foot to come into Leopard stance.

<u>Posture movement:</u>

With the feeling of continuing the circle from the previous movement, the right arm circles to the right and then over to finish palm facing outwards in front of the left shoulder. The left hand joins the right hand's circle to finish, palm away, to the left of the left shoulder – this position is often likened to a football goalkeeper saving a goal!

Move #29.

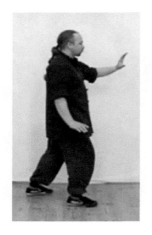 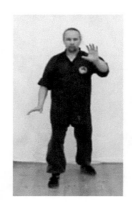

Stance: Right Dragon
Facing: East

<u>Stance movement:</u>

Step the right foot around and to the right, before transferring the weight into the right leg to come into a Dragon stance. Correct the left foot on the heel as the weight settles into the stance.

<u>Posture movement:</u>

The right hand circles down and across the front of the body to return to an 'active' position beside the right hip. The left hand 'pushes' forwards in an under-arm motion to finish extended in front of the left shoulder.

Move #30.

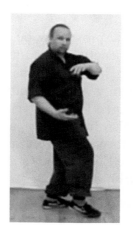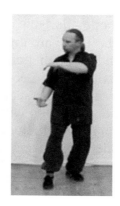

Stance: Right Cat
Facing: East

Stance movement:

Transfer the weight back into the left leg and draw the right foot in before lifting the heel into Cat stance.

Posture movement:

The left hand rolls to palm downwards to form a 'ball' with the right hand which simultaneously 'scoops' to palm upwards. The body is turned to the right from the waist so that the 'ball' is held to the right side of the body and the head is turned slightly further to the right to look to the rear.

Afterword:
A comment from the author.

I hope that this book proves to be helpful in your training. There are great benefits and a lot of enjoyment to be found through training in these Arts. The depth and complexity of the Lee Family Arts are truly staggering and have kept my interest engaged for many years.

I hope that you will also find benefit and pleasure from your training and I look forward to continuing my journey alongside you, beyond 'the Edge of the Cyclone'!

Conrad Robinson, 2017.

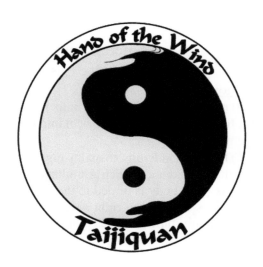

Notes:

Notes:

Notes